Healthy Choices 3

I0484151

Understanding the Thyroid and Endocrine System

Sheila K. Miles, N.D.,
N.H.S.D.
2015

Disclaimer

The health and nutrition information contained in this book is for educational purposes only. It is not meant to replace the advice of a medical professional.

Healthy Choices 3
Understanding the Thyroid and Endocrine System

By Sheila K. Miles, N.D., N.H.S.D.

Copyright 2015 by Sheila Miles
Edited by Roxanne Faison

ISBN-13: 978-1506133423

ISBN-10: 1506133428

To purchase Dr. Miles' books or eBooks go to
Amazon.com
http://www.drsheilamiles.com
http://www.choosing-natural-health.com

Contact Dr. Miles at
drsheilamiles@hotmail.com

Healthy Choices 3

Understanding the Thyroid and Endocrine System

Healthy Choices 3 –
Understanding the Thyroid and Endocrine System

Table of Contents

Introduction

As a Naturopath, the most common ailment that I see in my practice is a disorder with the endocrine system. I have written this book to try to clear up the functions of the different glands and their impact on the body.

I am not surprised that this is so prevalent. When we look at our food and water supply it is easy to understand why. The food is over processed and may be genetically modified, making it not even real food anymore. Our water is full of chemicals, such as fluoride, which is very hard on the thyroid. We are bombarded on every side and corner. Our body doesn't recognize this stuff as food and doesn't know how to process it. Therefore, it takes its toll on our glands and our entire body.

With a few modifications in diet and the addition of high quality supplements we can make a difference in how we feel and how our body functions.

Let's start our journey.......

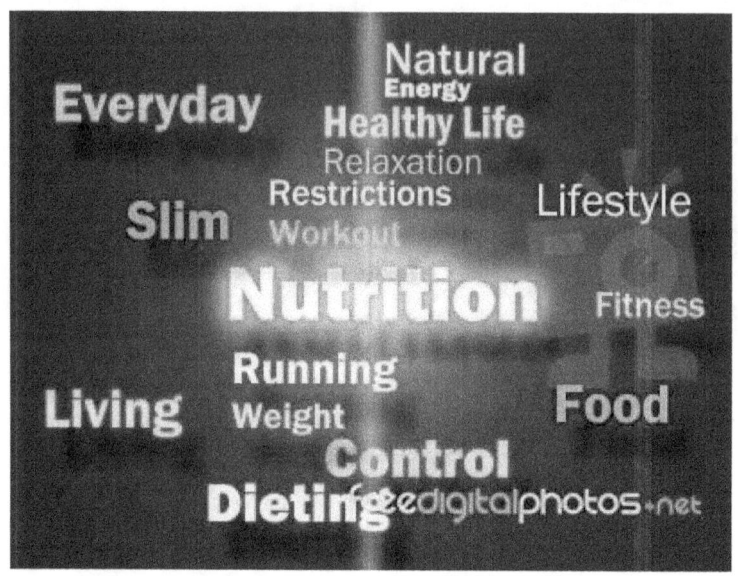

Healthy Choices 3
Understanding the Thyroid and
Endocrine System

Chapter 1

The Endocrine System

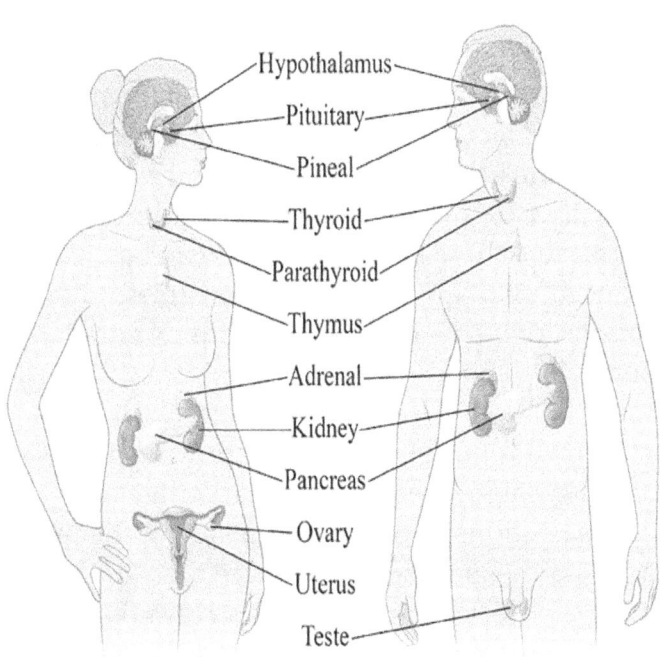

Hypothalamus
Pituitary
Pineal
Thyroid
Parathyroid
Thymus
Adrenal
Kidney
Pancreas
Ovary
Uterus
Teste

THE ENDOCRINE SYSTEM

We need to take a look at the entire endocrine system to fully understand how all of the glands function. They work together as a whole. So, it is a good idea to understand each gland and its function.

The endocrine system is a system of glands that produce and secrete hormones. These hormones regulate the body's growth, metabolism, sexual development, and function. They are chemical messengers which are created by the body. Hormones transfer information and instructions from one set of cells to another. You have many different hormones circulating in the bloodstream and each one affects only the cells that are genetically programmed to receive and respond to its message. These hormone levels can be influenced by many factors such as stress, infections, or even changes in the fluids and minerals in the body.

Some types of glands are specific such as the exocrine glands, sweat and salivary, they only release secretions in the skin or inside of the mouth. The endocrine glands release more than 20 hormones directly into the bloodstream that are then transported to cell in other parts of the body.

The major glands that make up the endocrine system are the hypothalamus, pituitary, thyroid, parathyroids, adrenals, pineal body, and the reproductive organs (ovaries and testes). The pancreas is also a part of this system, actually it has two purposes. It produces and secretes digestive enzymes, which makes it a part of the digestive system as well.

The above glands are the main hormone producers but some non-endocrine organs such as the brain, heart, lungs, kidneys, liver, thymus, skin, and placenta will also produce and release hormones.

HYPOTHALAMUS

Located in the lower central part of the brain you will find the hypothalamus gland. This is the part of the brain that regulates satiety, metabolism, and body temperature. The hypothalamus is the main link between the endocrine and nervous systems. The pituitary gland is controlled by the nerve cells in the hypothalamus with chemicals that are produced, which either stimulate or suppress the hormone secretions from the pituitary.

PITUITARY

The pituitary gland is no bigger than a pea and is located at the base of the brain just beneath the hypothalamus. It is considered the most important part of the endocrine system and is often called the "master gland". It produces hormones that control several other endocrine glands. The pituitary relies on the hypothalamus to relay information that is sensed by the brain such as temperature, feelings, and light exposure. Based on this information the pituitary will produce and secrete hormones.

The pituitary is divided into two parts, the anterior lobe and the posterior lobe. The anterior lobe regulates activity of the thyroid, adrenals, and reproductive glands. The posterior lobe controls the body's water balance by releasing anti-diuretic hormones. It also releases hormones to contract the uterus during childbirth and will stimulate the production of milk.

THYROID

The thyroid gland is located in the lower front part of the neck. The hormones produced here regulate the body's metabolism. They also play a role in bone growth and the development of the brain and nervous system in children. The release of these thyroid hormones is controlled by the pituitary. These hormones help to maintain normal blood pressure, heart rate, digestion, muscle tone, and reproductive functions.

PARATHYROID

Attached to the thyroid, on either side, are two pairs of tiny glands called the parathyroid. These glands regulate the level of calcium in the blood and bones.

ADRENAL GLANDS

The adrenals are two triangular-shaped glands that are located on top of each kidney. Each gland is made up of two parts. The outer part is called the adrenal cortex and the inner part is called the adrenal medulla. The adrenal cortex produces hormones that are called corticosteroids. These hormones regulate salt and water balance in the body, the body's metabolism, the immune system, how well the body handles stress, and sexual function. The inner part or the adrenal medulla produces adrenaline. These hormones increase the heart rate and blood pressure whenever the body is under stress.

PINEAL BODY

The pineal body or gland is located in the middle of the brain. It secretes the hormone melatonin. Melatonin is known for regulating the sleep-wake cycle.

GONADS OR REPRODUCTIVE GLANDS

These glands are the main source of sex hormones. In males, the testes secrete hormones, most importantly testosterone. Testosterone, along with the other hormones, affect male characteristics as well as sperm production. In women, the ovaries produce eggs and secrete the female hormones estrogen and progesterone. Estrogen controls the female characteristics and both hormones are involved in pregnancy and the regulation of the menstrual cycle. Progesterone balances and counteracts the adverse effects that estrogen can have. For instance, some women can produce too much estrogen, which increases the risk of breast and uterus cancer. Adding additional progesterone has been known to help with abnormal uterine bleeding, as well as pregnancy loss or premature labor.

THYMUS

The thymus is located in front of the heart beneath the breastbone. It is mainly composed of lymphatic tissue. Its purpose is to regulate the immune system. When we are younger our thymus gland is quite large and very active. It produces T-lymphocytes or T-cells, which are specific white blood cells that protect the body from viruses and infections. It also produces and secretes thymosin, which is a hormone necessary for T-cell development and production.

The thymus is not designed to last a lifetime. As we age, the thymus gland shrinks and by old age it is usually just composed of fat and fibrous tissues. Fortunately, the thymus produces all of your T-cells by puberty.

PANCREAS

The pancreas is located at the back of the abdomen behind the stomach. It has both digestive and hormonal functions. One part of the pancreas secretes digestive enzymes and the other part secretes hormones such as insulin and glucagon. These are the hormones that regulate the level of glucose or sugar in the blood.

PROBLEMS WITH THE ENDOCRINE SYSTEM

Too much or too little of any hormone can be harmful to the body. As an example, one of the hormones that the pituitary gland produces is growth hormone. If too much is produced you may grow too tall, if too little is produced you may be very short.

Adrenal Insufficiency - you may experience weakness, fatigue, skin changes, weight gain that is difficult to lose, or you may lose the ability to cope with stress.

Diabetes - when the pancreas fails to produce enough insulin then diabetes will occur. Symptoms include excessive thirst, weight loss, and hunger. If this condition occurs in children and teens, it is usually an autoimmune disorder in which specific immune cells and antibodies which are produced by the immune system attack and destroy the cells of the pancreas that produce insulin. This is known as Type 1 diabetes. It can cause long-term complications such as kidney problems, blindness, nerve damage, and even heart attack and stroke.

Type 2 diabetes occurs when the body cannot produce enough insulin or the body does not use it as it should. This is the most common form of diabetes. Obesity tends to be a risk factor in the onset of this form of diabetes.

Hyperthyroidism and Hypothyroidism –

Hyperthyroidism is a condition where the levels of thyroid hormone are very high. Symptoms include weight loss, nervousness, increased heart rate, and blood pressure, protruding eyes, and a swelling in the neck from an enlarged thyroid gland, known as a goiter.

Hypothyroidism occurs when there is too little thyroid hormone. Symptoms include fatigue, slow heart rate, dry skin, weight gain, and constipation. The most common cause of hypothyroidism in kids is a condition known as "Hashimoto's thyroiditis" or "Hashimoto's Disease". This occurs from an autoimmune process that damages the thyroid and blocks thyroid hormone production.

Chapter 2

Function of the Thyroid Gland

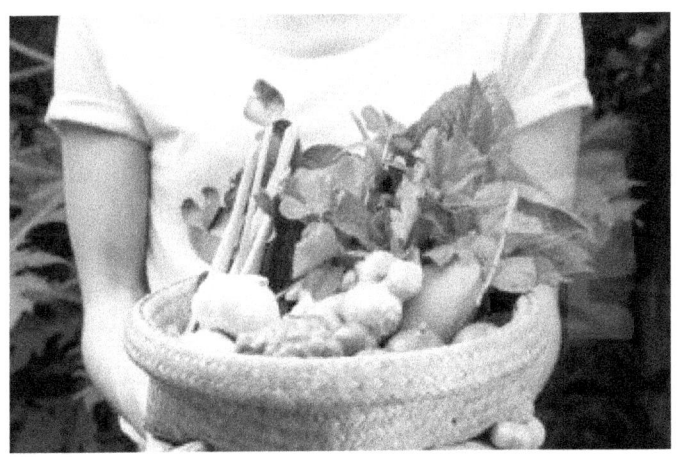

One of the more common problems that I see in my practice is hypothyroidism, usually paired with hypoadrenalism. These two problems can cause a myriad of symptoms ranging from acne to autoimmune dysfunction.

Obviously, you may suspect that you have one of these problems, or you wouldn't be reading this book. So let's start at the very beginning.

WHAT IS THE FUNCTION OF MY THYROID?

The thyroid is a butterfly shaped gland that is located in the lower part of the neck. Every muscle, organ, and cell depends on the production of adequate thyroid hormones for optimal functioning. These hormones also act as the body's metabolic regulator. If you are in a hypothyroid state, your thyroid is not releasing enough hormones to meet your body's demands and your metabolic rate is reduced. If you are in a hyperthyroid state, the thyroid is releasing an excess amount of hormones and you have an elevated metabolic rate. In the course of an entire year, the thyroid secretes approximately one teaspoon of hormones. This one tiny teaspoon will drive the metabolic rate of every cell in the body.

Symptoms of Hypothyroidism include the following:

Brittle nails
Hoarseness

Brain fog (inability to concentrate)
Hypotension
Cold hands and feet (cold intolerance)
Infertility
Constipation
Irritability
Depression
Muscle Cramps
Difficulty Swallowing
Muscle Weakness
Dry Skin
Nervousness
Elevated Cholesterol
Poor memory
Fatigue
Puffy eyes
Hair Loss
Slower heartbeat
Menstrual Irregularity
Throat pain
Weight gain

Hypothyroidism is probably one of the most prevalent conditions today. Approximately 13 million adults (probably more) have an undiagnosed hypothyroid condition. Blood tests are not reliable when testing the thyroid. They only take a picture of what is going on at that exact point in time. If you are on a thyroid supplement, a blood test is measuring what is circulating in the blood stream, not what the thyroid is actually picking up and using.

As a naturopath, I use the laboratory test, basal body temperature, hair analysis, and the client's signs and symptoms to determine the function of the gland.

The thyroid gland produces 2 major hormones. Thyroxine (T4) and Triiodothyronine (T3). These two hormones help the cells produce energy. If there are inadequate amounts of thyroid hormone produced (hypothyroidism) then the metabolism of the cells slows down and the signs and symptoms of hypothyroidism will be present. The thyroid produces more T4 (80%) than T3 (20%). T3 is more active than T4 and T3 is the hormone that increases the metabolism inside the cells. Most of the T4 is converted into T3 in the cells of the body.

The thyroid gland is stimulated by a hormone produced by the pituitary known as TSH or thyroid stimulating hormone. When TSH is secreted by the pituitary gland, it causes the thyroid gland to release thyroid hormones. T4 and T3 are very sensitive to TSH and whenever the body has adequate amounts of thyroid hormone available, the TSH levels are lowered, which lowers the production of the thyroid hormone.

DIAGNOSIS?

Conventional diagnosis consists of a blood test which primarily measures TSH. Physicians believe that if the TSH is normal that automatically rules out hypothyroidism. If the TSH is elevated, they believe that it is a sign that the pituitary gland is sensing a low thyroid hormone level in the body and the TSH is being secreted to stimulate the thyroid gland to produce more thyroid hormone, thus, hypothyroidism.

Normal range for TSH is 0.4-4.5 mIU/L. Hypothyroidism would be indicated if your range is greater than 4.5 mIU/L. Unfortunately, mis-diagnosis is common. If your lab tests are normal you might be sent home with an anti-depressant or just told "you are fine."

Thyroid physiology is very complex. The production, conversion, and the uptake of thyroid hormones in the body involve several steps. If there is a malfunction in any of these steps you can have hypothyroid symptoms, but these symptoms may not necessarily show up on any lab tests.

A standard blood thyroid panel usually only tests TSH and T4, typically not T3. These ranges can vary depending on the lab the physician is using. Lab ranges are set by averages of people who are being tested. Typically, sick people are the only ones who get tested, so are our "normal" ranges really normal? Not just on thyroid testing, but for any testing.

WHAT CAN GO WRONG?

1.   *Pituitary Dysfunction*

The pituitary gland is located at the base of the brain, near the hypothalamus. This tiny gland is the control center for all of the glands. It controls the thyroid and the adrenal glands.

If you have an active infection, blood sugar imbalances, chronic stress, pregnancy, hypoglycemia, or insulin resistance; this elevates cortisol, which causes the pituitary to become fatigued. When this happens it can no longer signal the thyroid to release enough thyroid hormone. So the thyroid gland itself may be perfectly normal, it just isn't receiving the right messages.

2.   *Conversion problems*

This is probably the most common problem with the thyroid. T4 is the inactive form of thyroid hormone and must be converted to T3 before it can be used by the body. This conversion can be halted by:

Chronic illness
Cigarette smoking

Drugs (propranolol, birth control pills, estrogens, lithium, methimazole, propylthiouracil, dexamethasone)
Growth hormone deficiency
Heavy metal toxicity
High stress
Low Adrenal states
Malnutrition
Mineral and vitamin deficiencies (selenium, vitamins A, B6, and B12)
Old age
Soy products
Elevated cortisol levels,
Inflammation

If you have a conversion problem, you will have hypothyroid symptoms but your TSH and T4 will be normal. If you have your T3 tested, it will be low.

3.   *Elevated TBG*

The protein that carries the thyroid hormone through the blood is called thyroid binding globulin (TBG). When thyroid hormone is bound to TBG, it is inactive and is unavailable to the tissues. When the TBG levels are high, levels of "free" thyroid hormone will be low, causing hypothyroid symptoms.

TSH and T4 will be normal in a blood test, T3 will be low, and T3 uptake and TBG will be high.

Elevated TBG can be caused by high estrogen levels. In order to bring this into balance, the estrogen must be cleared from the body.

4.   Decreased TBG

This is the opposite of the pattern above. Whenever your levels of TBG are low, levels of the "free" thyroid hormone will be high. Too much free thyroid hormone in the bloodstream will cause the cells to become resistant to it. There may be more than enough thyroid hormone, but the cells can't use it, therefore, you have hypothyroid symptoms.

TSH and T4 will be normal, T3 will be high and T3 uptake and TBG will be low.

This can be caused by high testosterone levels. It can be associated with polycystic ovary syndrome (PCOS) and metabolic syndrome. Restoring sugar balance is the key to treating this problem.

5.   Thyroid Resistance

In this case both the thyroid and the pituitary glands are working normally, but the hormones just aren't getting into the cells. All lab tests will be normal.

This is usually caused by chronic stress and high cortisol levels. It can also be caused by high homocysteine and genetic factors.

This is only a partial list of things that can go wrong. The physicians believe that one drug treats all, but each person is different and each case needs to be looked at differently. Synthroid, the drug of choice, is a synthetic hormone, which the body often does not recognize. This is not a "one pill cures all".

Healthy Choices 3
Understanding the Thyroid and
Endocrine System

Chapter 3

Hyperthyroidism

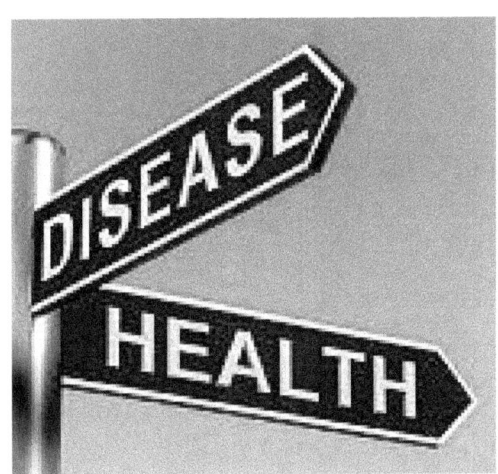

HYPERTHYROIDISM

So far, we have only discussed hypothyroidism, which is the secretion of too little thyroid hormone, but the opposite of that, is hyperthyroidism which can be just as bad, if not worse.

Symptoms of hyperthyroidism include:

Nervousness
Sweating
Heart palpitations
Nerve tingling
Fatigue
Heat intolerance
Hyperactivity
Eye disorders
Increased appetite
Goiter
Hypertension
Menstrual Disturbance
Weakness
Weight Loss

Hyperthyroidism can be caused by certain illnesses, most of which are autoimmune. An autoimmune disorder is a condition whereby the immune system malfunctions and produces antibodies against its own tissues. When working properly, the immune system is our body's defense mechanism against infection. Whenever we are attacked by bacteria, or some other foreign invader, the immune system fights the infection. It produces antibodies, which bind to the foreign substance and neutralize the infection.

Graves' disease and Hashimoto's disease are both autoimmune disorders of the thyroid gland. In both of these conditions the immune system produces antibodies which attack the thyroid gland. They can cause inflammation and possibly destruction of the gland. As the gland becomes more inflamed, it will release excess thyroid hormone. Thus, the signs of hyperthyroidism.

Autoimmune disorders are very prevalent. They are the leading cause of death in American women under age 65, affecting approximately 5% of women in the US. Women typically are diagnosed more frequently with these conditions than men.

Some common autoimmune disorders are:

Crohn's
Graves' disease
Hashimoto's
Juvenile Arthritis and Diabetes
Lupus
Multiple Sclerosis
Rheumatoid Arthritis
Scleroderma
Ulcerative Colitis
Chronic Fatigue Syndrome
Gulf War Syndrome

No one really knows why you develop an autoimmune disorder and conventional medicine is not very effective. Generally, they only treat the symptoms, not the true illness.

One of the ways to treat hyperthyroidism is to take a good look at the diet. You would need to avoid all stimulating substances, such as caffeine. In extreme cases, doctors give you a radioactive substance which kills the gland and then put you on hormones for the rest of your life. Because of the relationship between autoimmune disorders and hyperthyroidism, it is much more difficult to treat than hypothyroidism.

Chapter 4

The Adrenal Gland

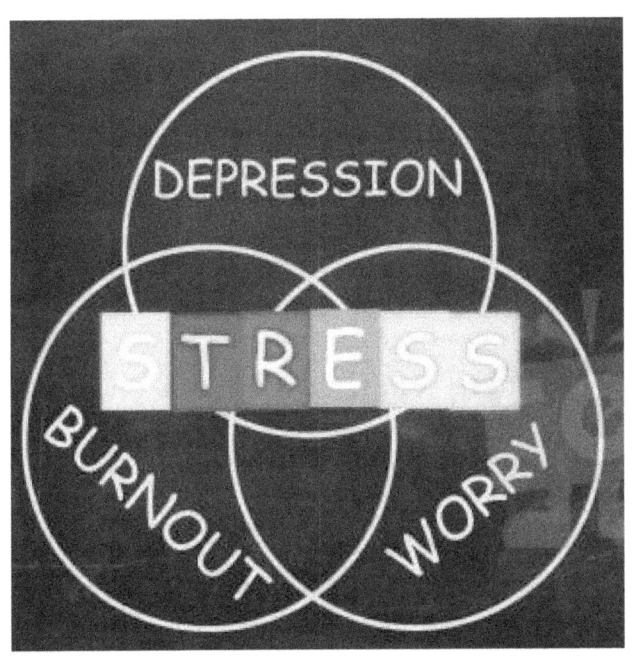

ADRENAL GLAND DYSFUNCTION

Are you tired all the time? Have difficulty losing weight? Your problem could be your adrenal glands. Just what are your adrenal glands and what do they do? Let's take a look.

The adrenal glands are small glands, which are located on top of your kidneys, they are also known as the "fight or flight" glands. Each one is about 3 inches wide and about ½ inch tall. These glands consist of three different regions. Each of these regions produces different hormones. Some of the hormones produced include DHEA, hydro-cortisone, estrogen, testosterone, progesterone, and pregnenolone. Each of these hormones interact with the thyroid hormone in the body. If the secretion of any of these hormones becomes inadequate, then you may have problems converting T4.

Some symptoms of adrenal gland dysfunction include:

- Fatigue and exhaustion
- Craving for salty and sweet foods
- Sleep that doesn't refresh (you get sleep, but wake up tired)
- Insomnia
- Unable to cope with stress
- Difficulty concentrating or brain fog
- Poor digestion
- Sensitivity to cold

- Allergies
- Low or high blood pressure
- You may feel more energetic in the evening
- Low immune function and slow recovery from illness or stress
- Muscle loss
- Belly fat
- Water retention
- Reduced sex drive
- Unable to remember things
- Constipation.

The hormones that the adrenals produce help to balance your blood sugar, which controls your energy. Each time your blood sugar drops, the adrenals will release hormones and cause the blood sugar to rise, which increases energy. They also release hormones when you are under stress. Our sympathetic nervous system takes over, basically our "fight or flight" system and stress hormones, such as adrenaline, norepinephrine, and cortisol are secreted. These hormones increase the heart rate and give you a surge of energy to prepare for the "emergency". Cortisol helps to maintain the blood pressure and fluid balance, but dwelling on your problems will cause cortisol to be continuously produced and can lead to a suppressed immune system, high blood pressure, blood sugar, obesity, acne, and much more.

If your adrenal glands are exhausted, all the rules of weight loss are reversed. Calorie restriction and exercise may make you fatter due to cortisol. Cortisol is secreted by the adrenals when you are under stress. This hormone is not your friend. It acts as a fat storing, muscle destroying, skin wrinkling, and age-accelerating enemy. Not only that, but it will cause you to retain fluid, making you feel even fatter. The areas of the body that have the greatest amount of cortisol receptors are your midsection, face, and upper back – let me guess – this is where most of your fat is accumulating.

Adrenal fatigue has been recognized, written about and treated for over a hundred years. Thousands of doctors have dealt with it and treated it, but it is not taught in medical schools today. Your average physician is unaware of its presence and seldom looks for it. Even an endocrinologist (a specialist who treats disorders of the glands) will rarely recognize adrenal fatigue as a condition and they not prepared to treat it. A cardiologist once told me that the adrenal glands were the most useless thing in the human body! You must become informed yourself. Low adrenal function is just one of those problems that have become invisible to modern medicine, with one exception, Addison's disease.

Addison's disease (hypoadrenia or the complete shut-down of the adrenal glands) and Cushing's disease (extremely high levels of cortisol mostly caused by steroid drugs) are both covered in medical texts, but adrenal fatigue is rarely, if ever, mentioned. The only tests that your doctor will run to detect hypoadrenia (low adrenal function) are the tests for Addison's disease. Most doctors won't even run these tests because they can be complicated to run and according to the medical profession the symptoms are vague and the condition is difficult to diagnose.

JUST WHAT IS ADRENAL FATIGUE?

Adrenal fatigue is any decrease in the ability of the adrenal glands to carry out their normal function. The main symptom is fatigue. The adrenals are unable to continue to properly respond to stress.

WHO SUFFERS FROM ADRENAL FATIGUE AND WHAT CAUSES ADRENAL FATIGUE?

Anyone of any age can suffer from adrenal fatigue. The adrenals can be weak from birth. If the mother has weak adrenals or the child experiences stress in the womb, they can have lowered adrenal function. C-section babies also tend to have lowered adrenal function because of stress and not passing through the birth canal. So from birth on, their ability to cope with stress can be diminished.

Babies with low adrenal function tend to be fussy and cry a lot. Older children can be sick more often and take longer to recover from illnesses.

Anyone who is under serious or repeated stress – injury, illness, allergies, inadequate nutrition, or just exposed to a toxic environment are also candidates for adrenal fatigue.

There are thousands of individual causes for adrenal fatigue but usually they stem from four common sources.

1.   Disease – such as cancer, bronchitis, AIDS, auto-immune.

2.   Physical stress – surgery, poor nutrition, exhaustion, etc.

3.   Emotional stress – relationships, work, or psychological stress.

4.   Continual and/or severe environmental stress. This could be from toxic pollutants in the air, water, or food.

CAN I RECOVER FROM ADRENAL FATIGUE?

Yes, if you receive the proper treatment, you can fully recover.

CAN ADRENAL FATIGUE AFFECT THE THYROID GLAND?

Yes, if one gland is tired, usually the others are also. They have to work harder to pick up the slack so they are also stressed.

Approximately 80% of the people who suffer from adrenal fatigue have some form of decreased thyroid function. These are typically the people who don't respond well to thyroid therapy. Generally, they are suffering from adrenal fatigue as well. If these people are to get well, the adrenals must be supported along with the thyroid.

MORE INFECTIONS? ANKLE SWELLING? ALLERGIES?

Adrenal function goes hand in hand with your immune function. If adrenal fatigue is present then you may have more respiratory infections – bronchitis and pneumonia.

One of the causes of ankle swelling is adrenal fatigue. There are other causes of ankle swelling so be sure to check your other symptoms and see if it is adrenal fatigue or some other disorder.

Allergies are more pronounced in someone with adrenal fatigue. Cortisol is the main hormone produced by the adrenals and is a strong anti-inflammatory substance. When this hormone drops, it becomes more likely that you will have an allergic (inflammatory) response and these allergic responses can be more severe.

ARE THERE ANY LABORATORY TESTS TO DETECT ADRENAL FATIGUE?

Yes, both saliva and hair analysis will detect adrenal fatigue. Saliva will tell what is going on at that point in time. A hair analysis looks at what has been going on with your body for the past month or so. It shows all of your mineral levels and gives perspective on which supplements you may need to boost the glands. Personally, I like the hair analysis better than saliva because I think it gives a more complete picture.

I SUFFER FROM FIBROMYALGIA, DEPRESSION, OR CHRONIC FATIGUE SYNDROME – COULD THIS BE RELATED TO ADRENAL FATIGUE?

Yes, adrenal fatigue is a common component in all of these problems.

HOW DO I TREAT ADRENAL FATIGUE?

First of all, you would need a test to determine the degree to which the adrenals are fatigued. Then we use targeted nutritional supplements. These supplements are specific vitamins/minerals/amino acids, which are formulated with ingredients to benefit the glands. I also like to use glandular extracts to rebuild these glands. One of the best products I have found for the glands is GTA from Biotics. GTA contains porcine glandular concentrate, along with a few other ingredients, and can do wonders for the thyroid. The glands can be rebuilt and you will feel better. It may take some time, but you didn't develop this problem overnight.

WHAT CAN I DO TO KEEP MY ADRENALS HEALTHY?

Just simply follow the overall principles of good health. Eat high quality food, get regular exercise, and rest. Try to keep a good mental attitude. If you are under stress, which most of us are at some point in our lives, then you may need to add nutritional supplements to keep your adrenal glands healthy.

Here is a questionnaire to help determine if you may have adrenal fatigue.

For any symptom you have experienced in the last month, mark with a YES

My life is very stressful. _____
I am easily startled and suffer from panic attacks. ____

I feel tired but wired. ___
I often feel weak and shaky. ___
When I stand up quickly, I feel dizzy. ___

I have dark circles under my eyes. ___

I crave sweets. ___

I crave salt. ___

I don't feel refreshed after a night's sleep. ___

I have difficulty either falling asleep
or staying asleep. ___

I have trouble concentrating or suffer
from mental fogginess. ___

I frequently experience headaches. ___

I catch colds easily and suffer from
frequent infections. ___

I can't start my day without caffeine. ___

I retain water. ___

I experience heart palpitations. ___

I have poor tolerance for alcohol, caffeine,
and other drugs. ___

I don't tolerate exercise well and I'm
incredibly tired afterwards. ___

I have hypoglycemia (low blood sugar). ___

My muscles are weak. ___

My blood pressure is low. ___

I am sensitive to bright light (need to wear
sunglasses when outside). ___

If you answered yes to 0-7 you may have a low
adrenal dysfunction.
8-10 moderate adrenal dysfunction
11 or more – severe adrenal dysfunction.

Healthy Choices 3
Understanding the Thyroid and Endocrine System

Chapter 5

Hormones

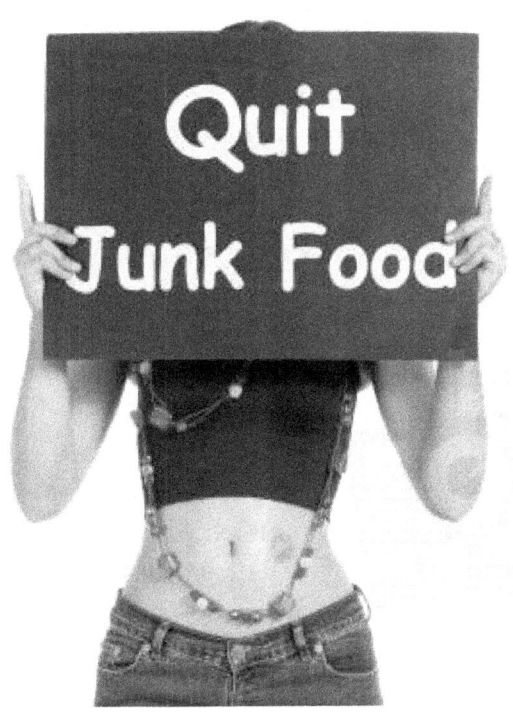

HORMONES

DHEA

DHEA (dehydroepiandrosterone) is produced in the adrenal glands. This hormone, which is a steroid, peaks at an early age and fades as we age. It can have a protective effect against Cardiovascular Disease, Obesity, Hyperhcolesterol, Cancer, Lupus, Diabetes, and certain other autoimmune illnesses. Most people who have a chronic disease, such as Rheumatoid Arthritis, Cancer, MS, Crohn's, and Chronic Fatigue Syndrome, typically have low levels.

There is a relationship between low levels of DHEA and hypothyroidism. Whenever you treat the thyroid, it works better if you use a combination of thyroid hormone and DHEA, rather than using each individually. However too much DHEA can reverse this effect, so it is best to start with low doses.

Anyone who has a chronic illness should have their DHEA levels checked. Side effects from too much are rare but can produce headache, fatigue, insomnia, and congestion. DHEA affects hormone levels, so it can cause other symptoms. Women may have abnormal periods or mood changes. They could also take on masculine characteristics, such as facial hair or a deeper voice. Men might develop more breast tissue, high blood pressure, or other problems. Remember, these are rare.

HYDROCORTISONE

Hydrocortisone is produced in the adrenal glands, just like DHEA. This hormone is the body's main defense against stressful situations, including infections and injuries. When this hormone has an increase in production, you are more susceptible to illnesses. If you have deficient hydrocortisone production, a replacement can improve the immune system and may reverse many chronic conditions without serious side effects. However, the high doses given in conventional medicine will not produce these positive effects.

The possible side effects which are associated with hydrocortisone, as with any steroid, are weight gain, osteoporosis, arteriosclerosis, and abnormalities with blood sugar. Typically, if you use doses of less than 40 mg per day there will be no major side effects.

TESTOSTERONE

Testosterone is also produced in the adrenal glands. Although many consider this to be just a male hormone, women also produce this hormone. Its production fades as we age which can cause a loss of sex drive in both men and women.

Testosterone levels are usually low in hypothyroid men, as these two conditions seem to go hand in hand.

Some symptoms of low testosterone in men are:

Decreased sex drive
Erectile dysfunction
Reduced energy level
Reduced strength and endurance levels
Sleep problems
Emotional problems including sadness, irritability,
        difficulty concentrating, and depression
Increased breast size and tenderness
Hair loss

More serious

Obesity
Heart Attack and Strokes
Diabetes
Metabolic Syndrome

It is always a good idea for both men and women to have your levels checked.

Normal levels for men:

Age 25	700
Age 35	650
Age 45	600
Age 55	550
Age 65	500
Age 75	450
Age 85	400

Conventional medical practitioners are reluctant to treat low testosterone in men or women because of process called aromatization. This is a process by which the body will convert excess testosterone into estrogen. The body is trying to keep a balance between male and female hormones in the body. Males have natural amounts of the female hormones estrogen and progesterone, but what makes the difference is that they don't have hundreds or thousands of milligrams of testosterone just floating around. The average male produces about 7mg of testosterone per day. That is about fifty milligrams per week. The weakest injectable testosterone you can find is fifty milligrams and most doctors won't use it because it is too weak. So they use very large doses and since the body likes balance, the estrogen goes up. Now, if the estrogen stays in proportion to the testosterone, you don't have much cause for worry, but if you produce an enzyme called aromatase, that could be a different story. Aromatase is an enzyme whose primary function is converting testosterone to estrogen. The more of this enzyme you have in your body, the more conversion you will have. Some estrogen is beneficial for men and not always a bad thing, but you can have too much of anything.

One of the ways to slow this conversion is to look at your diet. Eating snacks or meals that are loaded in carbohydrates, especially from refined, processed white flour and sugar will cause the highest surge in aromatase. You especially don't want to eat these high carb meals at night. Cut these out if you are trying to raise your testosterone.

Zinc is also an important mineral for keeping the aromatase enzyme at bay. Zinc also builds a strong immune and reproductive system. A simple way of testing your zinc levels is a "zinc taste test". I offer these tests in my office. You simply take a sip of liquid zinc, if you can taste it, your zinc levels are sufficient, if it has no taste, you need to supplement zinc. Never supplement zinc on your own for more than a month because it can deplete your copper.

There is an herbal flavonoid called Chrysin which has some preliminary lab research showing its ability to block the aromatization of testosterone to estrogen. Human studies are lacking, so validity of these results are questionable. The dosage would be 200-600 milligrams taken nightly with a meal.

By not treating this condition, medical practitioners are not taking into consideration the 50 studies that document the protective effects of testosterone against cardiovascular disease in men. The heart contains more testosterone receptors than any other muscle in the body. Men with angina who are given testosterone saw an improvement in symptoms and increased exercise tolerance, because the testosterone dilates the arteries of the heart.

Men who have suffered heart attacks have been shown to have low levels of testosterone and high levels of estrogen. I believe that any man with heart disease should have his testosterone levels checked and, if low, they should be restored to youthful levels. If the problem is hormone related, why use drugs to treat this problem?

Testosterone not only is effective in treating autoimmune thyroid disorders but also is effective in other disorders such as Lupus or Rheumatoid Arthritis. In these chronic illnesses you often have injured tissues, since testosterone is an anabolic (muscle building) hormone, it aids the body in repairing these tissues. Studies have been conducted showing that low levels of androgens, such as testosterone and DHEA have been thought to play a role in the development of autoimmune disease. *(Lahita, RG. "Increased oxidation of testosterone in systemic Lupus erythemaosis." Arthritis Rheum. 1983;26:1517-1521)*.

You need to keep the dosages of testosterone small so as to not shut off the body's own production of this hormone.

If you are looking for natural supplements to boost your levels there is an herb called Tribulus Terrestris. The dosage would be 200-750 mg per day. Look for products that contain about 20%

protodioscin, one of the most active components of tribulus. There is also homeopathic testosterone available in my office. This stimulates your body to produce more testosterone and eliminates the worry of aromatization.

As with all hormones, I recommend using the natural form of the hormone. When used appropriately, bio-identical testosterone is extremely safe and effective with no adverse effects. It is best to avoid treatment if the patient has had a diagnosis of prostate cancer. Also, you might add Saw Palmetto with any kind of testosterone treatment to avoid negative effects on the prostate. Saw Palmetto can reduce estrogen levels and prostate cancer is an estrogen driven cancer.

PROGESTERONE

Progesterone is one of the major hormones produced by the ovaries in females. Men produce very tiny amounts in the adrenal glands and the testicular glands. This hormone acts as a precursor for the adrenal hormones, which are estrogen, testosterone, and hydrocortisone.

You must have adequate amounts of thyroid hormones for the production of progesterone in the ovaries. This production can be disrupted by either hypothyroidism or hyperthyroidism.

Natural progesterone is available in a cream form as well as a pill form. The cream seems to work better than the pill form if you are using it for hormone balance. When the cream is rubbed into the skin it reaches all tissues, making it a reliable delivery system.

If you are using progesterone for insomnia or seizures then the pill form is better. When you take the progesterone pill it creates a metabolite allopregnanole in large amounts when progesterone is processed in the liver, this stimulates GABA receptors in the brain, which promotes relaxation and helps to balance the nervous system.

Be careful when buying the over the counter progesterone as the strengths can vary from jar to jar. Always make sure you buy from a reputable company.

Side effects can include breast tenderness, moodiness, and weight gain. These are rare and are usually dose related. You would simply lower the dose or slowly stop altogether. Side effects from the synthetic version (Provera) include breast cancer, blood clots, fluid retention, breast tenderness, nausea, insomnia, depression, and others. You are much safer with the natural form of this hormone.

ESTROGEN

Estrogen is primarily produced in the ovaries. There are different types of estrogen:

Estrone or E1 – usually measured after menopause or can be measured to test for cancer of the ovaries, testicles or adrenal glands.

Estrodiol or E2 – most commonly measured type of estrogen for non- pregnant women.

Estriol or E3 – usually only measured in pregnancy.

Estrogens are usually prescribed for the relief of hot flashes during menopause. They also slow down the rate of bone loss during the postmeno-pausal years and can help to improve memory loss in some patients.

There are numerous concerns about the use of estrogen treatment. There is a possible interaction of estrogen therapy and certain cancers, such as breast cancer. Although, this seems to be from the synthetic estrogen, we should be conservative in our use of any estrogen therapy.

Increased estrogen can lower the circulating thyroid hormone levels and can inhibit the conversion of T4 to T3. Birth control pills have been found to do this.

We seem to be living in a sea of estrogen. More and more people, men and women, are becoming estrogen dominate. We are constantly exposed to xenoestrogens in our environment - PCB's, Dioxins, and all sorts of chemicals. Hormones are added to a lot of our food. All of this can cause an estrogen dominate condition which could be responsible for the high rate of breast and prostate cancers. Try to limit your exposure to these chemicals and try to purchase organic, grass fed beef.

HUMAN GROWTH HORMONE

This hormone is secreted by the pituitary gland, located in the center of the brain. Its production peaks during adolescence. Children that lack the proper production of this hormone will have an extremely short stature. Adults will show signs of accelerated aging (increased wrinkles), decreased energy levels, low sexual function, body fat, osteoporosis, along with accelerated cardiovascular disease.

Our production of this hormone decreases as we age. Perhaps by supplementing HGH along with DHEA, testosterone, and the other hormones, we may slow down or in some instances, reverse aging. Maybe we might even lessen the symptoms of some chronic diseases such as Fibromyalgia, Arthritis, or Chronic Fatigue Syndrome.

The regulation and release of this hormone is regulated by thyroid hormones, so if you suffer from hypothyroidism it is a good possibility that your levels of human growth hormone are low. They are very closely related. Supplementation with growth hormone is very expensive. There are other ways to raise your levels:

1.   Exercise;
2.   Supplementation with other natural hormones;
3.   Supplementation with an amino acid complex;
4.   Gammanol Forte (a product from Biotics) was shown to raise growth hormone levels by over 45% in women. This was a study conducted by Dr. David Brownstein.

PREGNENOLONE

This hormone is a steroid hormone produced in the adrenal glands and is known as the "mother hormone". It is the precursor hormone to all of the adrenal glands. It is necessary to produce all other hormones and is formed from cholesterol.

Like all of the hormones, its production declines with age and is lower in individuals suffering from hypothyroidism. Combining this hormone with some thyroid hormone has been every effective. This combination helps patients recover energy and improve memory.

NATURAL HORMONES

When you use the natural hormones appropriately, they are very safe and effective. Before treatment, it is important to have a hormonal evaluation. This can be done using blood or saliva. Personally, I prefer blood. I think it is more accurate.

Small doses should be used and synthetic versions should be avoided if at all possible. Any hormone supplementation should be closely monitored by a qualified health care practitioner who understands their use. Hormones need to be in balance and it is best to use a combination rather than treating with individual hormones.

Chapter 6

Iodine

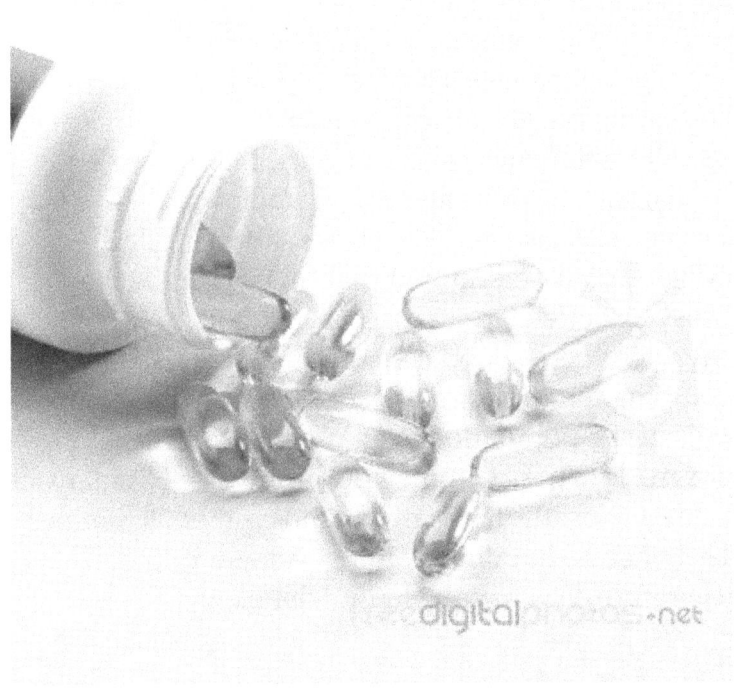

IODINE

Everybody associates iodine with the thyroid gland, but iodine does so much more. As a matter of fact, without iodine you could not live. It is found in each of the trillions of cells in our bodies. Not only does it work with the production of thyroid hormone, but production of all other hormones in the body. It is necessary for proper immune function and it is antibacterial, anti-parasitic, antiviral, and anticancer. It is also used in the treatment of fibrocystic breasts and ovarian cysts.

Most vitamins and minerals are present in food, but not so with iodine. If it is present in the soil, some may be absorbed into the food, but it is usually not in adequate amounts. Many ocean foods, such as fish and sea vegetables contain iodine. It is also added to table salt. The U.S. Government determined that this would be the most cost effective way to prevent goiter of the thyroid gland. Good idea, but table salt is just a combination of chemicals and probably less than 50% of the population even uses this chemical storm. Most of us in the know, now use Himalayan crystal sea salt. This salt contains minerals that our body needs, but does not have added iodine. Therefore, you may be iodine deficient.

Iodine is essential for all of the thyroid hormones. T4 (thyroxine) contains four iodine molecules and T3 (triiodothyronine) contains three iodine molecules. Without this iodine, the thyroid gland is unable to make the thyroid hormone in adequate amounts.

Deficiency of iodine can have many consequences. It can cause estrogen production to increase. This can lead to an increased sensitivity of breast tissue to estrogen. This increases your chance of developing diseases of the breast, including breast cancer. Fibrocystic breast disease responds well to iodine therapy.

In men, prostate cancer is similar to breast cancer in women, as it is an estrogen driven cancer. Iodine deficiency could be the link for the increased risk of this cancer in men.

The Recommended Daily Allowance for iodine is .150mg a day. However, since this was determined to be the amount to prevent goiter, it may not be adequate for optimum health. Without proper supervision, I would not recommend a larger dose. Too much iodine can actually harm the thyroid and may cause other symptoms, such as:

1. Allergy.
2. Autoimmune thyroid disease.
3. Detoxification reactions.
4. Iodine-induced hypothyroidism and goiter.

5. Iodine-induced hyperthyroidism.
6. Thyroid cancer.

Chapter 7

What Can We Do?

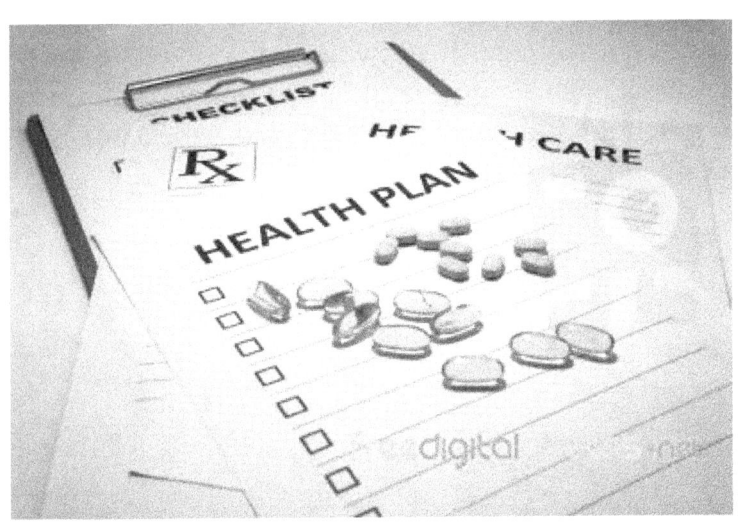

WHAT CAN WE DO?

One of the first things we need to look at with hypothyroidism or hyperthyroidism is our diet. Most diets consist of a lot of toxic elements. These include trans-fats, artificial sweeteners, GMO foods, and way too many chemicals. Whenever you are trying to heal from any kind of dis-ease you need a balanced, healthy diet, free from as many toxic substances as possible.

You are what you eat. Food is our fuel. It should furnish us with vitamins and minerals that our body can use. If we consume food that is refined or contains chemicals, the body must use its own supply of nutrients to break it down. If we don't have adequate supplies, then we are setting ourselves up for diseases. Just think what would happen to your car if you watered down your gas or added some foreign chemicals. It might run for a while but would eventually break down. Your body works the same way.

BASIC HEALTH GUIDELINES

Here are some guidelines to help keep you healthy and detoxified.

1. **Most Important** - drink water daily. Divide your weight by 2 and drink at least that amount in ounces daily. Make sure that it is from a pure source. *Never* drink tap water, because of the many chemicals they add to purify it. Your average tap water has been "flushed" about three times. Reverse osmosis is the purest form. Minimize liquids at meals; drink your water between meals.

2. Use a shower de-chlorinator and chlorine free dishwasher detergent to minimize your exposure to chlorine. You will also want to limit your exposure to bromine. Bromine is a common endocrine disrupter, meaning that it can inhibit thyroid hormone production causing a low thyroid state. This is in white bread, hot tubs and pools, along with some beverages.

3. Consume only organic fruits and vegetables and purchase them in quantities for quick consumption. Remember, fresh is best. Avoid peeling vegetables as the skin contains a lot of the nutrients. Try to eat your fruits and vegetables as near the natural state as possible. Cooking destroys nutrients.

4. Eat portions of mixed green salads and raw vegetables every day.

5. Eat fresh fruits in season. Try to stay with "what grows in your own backyard". Apples, plums, and pears are always good choices. Red apples are easier on the digestion.

6. Eat whole grains. Try quinoa, spelt, millet, and brown rice.

7. If you choose to drink milk, drink only organic milk.

8. Eat organic butter and healthy fats from olive oil, coconut oil, and avocados. Eliminate trans fats completely. Read your labels. Avoid the food if it contains the words "partially hydrogenated" or "shortening" in the ingredients list. Even if it says "zero trans fats" but "partially hydrogenated" or "shortening" are listed – trans fats are in that food. Under FDA regulations currently in effect in the United States, "if the serving contains less than 0.5 gram (of trans fat), the content, when declared, shall be expressed as zero." Look at that closer, for instance, if a product contains 0.4 grams of trans fat per serving and you eat 4 servings, you have just consumed 1.6 grams of trans fats, even though the package says zero.

9. Eat only organic meats and free range eggs. Avoid GMO (genetically modified organisms) foods. These foods have been artificially manipulated in a laboratory through genetic engineering. Most nations have banned the use of GMO foods while about 80% of foods here in America are genetically modified. There is growing evidence that GMOs cause many health issues, environmental damage, and are a violation of farmers' and consumers' rights.

10. Instead of reaching for a soda or a cup of coffee, drink herb teas and use stevia or some raw honey as a sweetener. Stevia is a natural herbal sweetener and contains no calories.

11. Avoid all artificial sweeteners. They are poison.

12. Bounce on a mini-trampoline for at least four or five minutes a day. This stimulates the movement of lymphatic fluids, which will help keep your body detoxed.

13. Get rid of the table salt. Celtic sea salt and Himalayan crystal salt are nourishing to the body instead of being toxic.

14. *No* high fructose corn syrup. This causes a non-alcoholic fatty liver disease. Not to mention that it is made from GMO corn.

15. Read labels. You would be surprised what is in your food when you start reading the labels. If you can't pronounce it, you probably don't need to be eating it.

16. You should be eating enough fiber rich foods that you have a bowel movement at least 2-3 times a day. If this is not you, you might want to consider a colon cleanse.

17. Each week pick one processed food and remove it from your diet. Replace it with a healthy food and before you know it, you will be eating a healthy diet.

Certain foods are hard on the thyroid and I have included a diet specific for hypothyroidism.

HYPOTHYROIDISM DIET

In order to increase the metabolic rate and raise energy production you should eat a high protein food at each meal. Lean protein is the best and should constitute about 40% of the total caloric value of each meal. Lean beef, fish and fowl are good sources. You might also include bean and grain combinations and eggs.

Increase frequency of meals…while decreasing the total caloric intake for each meal. This is suggested in order to sustain the level of nutrients necessary for energy production, and decrease blood sugar fluctuations.

You should eat a moderate amount of unrefined carbohydrates. Carbs should not exceed 40% of total daily calories. Good sources of unrefined carbohydrates would include whole grain products, legumes and root vegetables.

Avoid all sugars and refined carbohydrates... This includes white and brown sugar, honey, candy, soda pop, cake, pastries, alcohol and white bread. Sugars are very hard on the thyroid and the metabolic rate.

Keep your intake of fats and oils to about 20% of your total daily caloric intake. This would include fried foods, cream, butter, salad dressings, mayonnaise, etc.

Reduce or avoid milk and milk products....such as cheese, yogurt, ice cream, etc. These foods should be reduced to no more than once every three or four days. If you are suffering from hypothyroidism, we will assume that the parathyroid is also not functioning properly. The parathyroid gland determines where our calcium goes and if its function is decreased the calcium goes to the soft tissues (such as the gallbladder or kidneys) instead of the bones and teeth. If this calcium goes to the soft tissues you may be prone to kidney stones, hardening of the arteries, or gall stones. Gall stones are produced in the liver, so you can still have them even if you have had your gallbladder removed. Until this gland works properly, anything containing calcium should be avoided.

Reduce your fruit juice intake.....This includes orange juice, apple juice, grape juice and grapefruit juice. These juices help you to hold onto your calcium and they may also contain arsenic, particularly apple juice.

Here is a list of foods that may decrease thyroid activity, along with the metabolic rate and can cause numerous symptoms such as: fatigue, cold sensitivity, depression, weight gain, dry skin and hair, constipation, headaches, joint stiffness, water retention, and weight gain. You should avoid these foods until the function of the thyroid is restored.

Cabbage	Kale
Rutabagas	White Turnips

Cole Slaw
Sauerkraut
Soybeans
Chlorinated Water
Mustard
Swiss Cheese
Kale
Monterey Cheese
Mozzarella Cheese
Tortilla Roll
Almonds
Sardines
Hazelnuts
Torula Yeast
Parmesan Cheese
Dulse
Dandelion Greens
Mustard Greens

Flourides
Horseradish
Broccoli
Collards
Walnuts
Turnip Greens
Blue Cheese
Soybean Flour
Yogurt
American Cheese
Brewers Yeast
Cheddar Cheese
Kelp
Carob Powder
Pancake Mix
Cream

Avoid fats such as:

Salad Dressings
Cream
Hazelnuts
Margarine
Bockwurst
Salami
Bologna
Corn Chips
Bacon
Duck
Avocado
Cocoa Powder

Cheese (most)
Butter
Walnuts
Pork
Milk
Peanut Butter
Pork Links
Almonds
Knockwurst
Goose
Braunschweiger
Peanuts

Sardines (canned)
Tuna (canned in oil)
Avocado Oil
Liverwurst
Coconut Oil

These are just some of the basic foods to avoid. It is best to have a hair analysis, which will show all of your mineral levels. For instance, you may need more potassium rich foods, amino acids, or targeted vitamins.

HYPERTHYROIDISM DIET

If your thyroid is too fast you need to increase the intake of high purine protein foods such as liver, kidney and heart. Other good sources are sardines, tuna, clams, crab, lobster, and oysters. These types of protein should constitute about 33% of your daily calorie intake.

Typically, with a fast thyroid you burn all your calcium and magnesium quickly so you need to increase milk and milk products, all calcium rich foods, such as cheese, yogurt cream, and unsalted butter. Also increase the intake of nuts and seeds such as almonds, walnuts, peanuts, peanut butter and sunflower seeds. These foods which are high in fat should only constitute approximately 33% of your daily calorie intake.

Reduce your carbohydrate intake – including unrefined carbohydrates. Avoid cereals, whole grains and whole grain products. Carbohydrates should only constitute about 33% of your daily calorie intake.

Avoid all sugars and refined carbohydrates – all white and brown sugar, honey, candy, soda, cake, pastries, alcohol, and white bread.

Here is a list of foods that are high in magnesium and calcium; you should add more of these to your diet.

Blackstrap molasses
Prunes
Avocados
Bananas
Bass (broiled)
Figs (dried)

Corn
Cashews
Wild Rice
Tofu
Garbanzo Beans

Mozzarella Cheese
Milk
Monterey Cheese
Almonds
Swiss Cheese

Turnip Greens
Mustard Greens
Yogurt
Cream
Buttermilk

Calcium absorption is greatly enhanced when the diet is high in amino acids, such as Lysine, and Arginine. These proteins also help to reduce acidity of the tissues. Both effects are favorable for the fast metabolizer, so add the following foods to your diet.

Lima Beans	Salami
Garbanzo Beans	Sausage (lean)
Rump roast	Lamb
Skim Milk	Smelt
Beef Stew	Vegetable Stew
Cottage Cheese	Canadian Bacon
Spare ribs	Peanuts
Lentils	Bass
Flounder	Heart
Cod	Chuck roast
Ham	Liverwurst

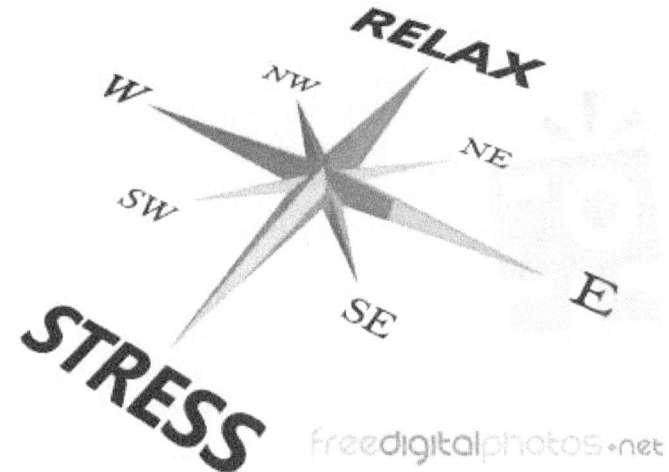

Healthy Choices 3
Understanding the Thyroid and Endocrine System

Chapter 8

Summing It All Up

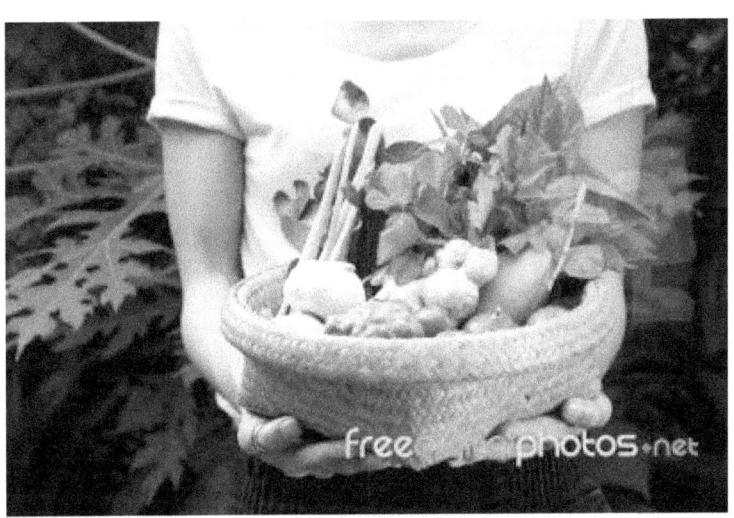

Whenever we have a hormone imbalance, our entire body feels out of whack. But with the proper diet, targeted supplements, and just a basic understanding of what is going on, we can make remarkable improvements in the way that we feel.

Remember, when we start treatment, we didn't get this way overnight and we are not going to heal overnight. So, be patient. There is no magic pill to correct these issues, but they can be healed.

My best advice to you is to educate yourself. You know your body better than anyone else. You are your best patient advocate. Use your knowledge and chose the correct path.

Stay Strong!

ABOUT THE AUTHOR

Dr. Sheila Miles is a native of South Central Kentucky, and grew up with a deep understanding of culture, tradition, and the many intangibles that make us who we are. She also saw close-to-hand a wide spectrum of health problems, and the ways country people had learned to deal with them, sometimes because a doctor was not available, and sometimes because the natural ways were better than the doctors'.

While coping with normal health issues involved in raising her own family, Sheila realized that she could help them better, and help her community as well, by learning more about natural medicine.

She went back to school, and in 2000 was Board Certified as a Naturopathic Physician by the National Board of Examiners in Integrated/Alternative Medicine and Natural Health Science. In addition, she earned a Doctorate in Natural Health Science.

Dr. Miles is certified in Iridology, Manipulation, Hydrotherapy, Acupressure Massage, Nutrition, Homeopathy, and Herbal Preparations.

Currently, she is working on her certification as a Life Coach and a NLP practitioner.

She feels a strong mission to help wherever possible, using the natural medical practices that work in harmony with our own systems to bring about natural health.